Glow Guide™
Yoga

II040587

Glow Guide™
Yoga

Simple Steps for Health and Well-Being

By Andrea McCloud

Illustrations by
Karen Greenberg

CHRONICLE BOOKS
SAN FRANCISCO

Text copyright © 2003 by Andrea McCloud.
Illustrations copyright © 2003 by Karen Greenberg.
Chronicle Books, the Chronicle Books eyeglasses logo and
Glow Guides are either registered trademarks or trademarks of
Chronicle Books LLC in the United States and/or other countries.
All rights reserved. No part of this book may be reproduced in
any form without written permission from the publisher.

Library of Congress Cataloging-in-Publication Data:

McCloud, Andrea.

Yoga : simple steps for health and well-being /
by Andrea McCloud ; illustrations by Karen Greenberg.
        p. cm. — (Glow guide)
Includes bibliographical references.
ISBN 0-8118-3809-9
1. Yoga—Health Aspects. I. Title. II. Series.
RA781.7 .M397 2003
613. 7'046—dc21
        2002014274

Manufactured in China

Designed by Greenberg Kingsley/NYC

Distributed in Canada by Raincoast Books
9050 Shaughnessy Street
Vancouver, British Columbia V6P 6E5

10 9 8 7 6 5 4 3 2 1

Chronicle Books LLC
85 Second Street
San Francisco, California 94105

www.chroniclebooks.com

Not all exercises are suitable for everyone. Your physical condition and health are important
factors in determining which yoga exercises, positions, and advice may be appropriate. This or
any other exercise program may result in injury. The author and publisher of this book disclaim
any liability from any injury that may result from the use, proper or improper, of any exercise
or advice contained in this book. Please consult your professional health care provider for information and advice on the suitability of your exercise program.

Dedication
To Derek, the quintessential yogi:
flexible, strong, and balanced.
Thank you.

- -

Acknowledgments
A big thanks to my friends and
family, who claimed never to tire
of hearing about yoga—and they
heard about it a lot—or seeing
me demonstrate my favorite
postures. Special thanks to my
editor, Mikyla, for being so
good at what she does, and to
the team at Chronicle Books, for
their hard work and dedication.

Introduction: The Yoga Glow

Glow is a beautiful luminance that comes from a balance of good mental and physical health, personal happiness, self-understanding, and self-confidence. You can't buy glow or wear glow; you can't apply it or borrow it from a friend. Glow comes from within. It's an inner radiance that is realized by taking care of yourself and being good to yourself. It's you at your best.

Turning a glimmer into a full-fledged glow isn't always easy, and it does take time and commitment. At the core of glow lies a healthy mind and body, and for many of us, those are things we must work for. But if you do the work, you reap the benefits. Simple as that. Not sure where to start? One word: yoga.

An ancient tradition deeply rooted in Indian and Hindu philosophy, yoga is the union of the mind, body, and soul, a balance of our intellectual, physical, and emotional sides. It's not a religion, nor is it simply an exercise regimen. Yoga is a commitment to health and well-being, a commitment to a better you.

No matter what your fitness level or degree of flexibility, or how coordinated or uncoordinated you may be, yoga can work for you. There's just one criterion: you've got to stick with it. Through the practice of *asanas* (postures) and *pranayama* (breath control), yoga works all of the muscle groups, stimulates the internal systems, and improves strength, flexibility, and balance, all the while calming the mind, reducing stress, and enhancing your inner and outer poise. Talk about a full-body workout!

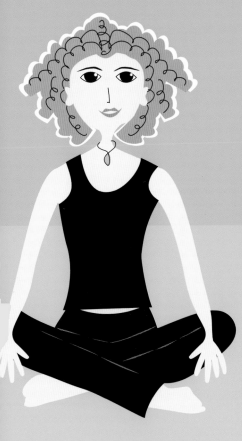

This book was designed to help you cultivate your yoga glow. It is divided into five sections: Strong Statements, Blissful Balancers, Essential Energizers, Meltdown Menders, and Blues Busters. Each section corresponds with what you might be needing from your yoga practice—strength, balance, energy, relaxation, rejuvenation—from day to day. You can do these poses anywhere and anytime. It's a good idea to first get comfortable with the more basic standing and balancing postures before you advance to the more difficult poses, but once you feel confident, jump around and experiment.

Choose one posture, do an entire section, or develop your own series (see Mixing It Up for a few important pointers)—whatever you can fit into your schedule. And remember, have fun and keep practicing!

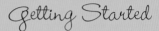
Getting Started

When to Practice and for How Long
When you're first starting, it's best to practice three to five days a week for fifteen to thirty minutes each time. When to practice really depends on your schedule and how much time you're willing to commit to yoga. Scan your calendar for time availability. Do you tend to work late? You'll probably want to practice in the morning. Can't get up early? Use your lunch hour. Whatever you decide, it's a good idea to be consistent and stick with a set schedule. This will help keep you motivated and practicing on a regular basis.

What to Wear
Wear something comfortable, nothing too tight or too loose, and go in bare feet. This will allow your feet to grip the floor and will help keep you from slipping. Your clothes should allow you to see the shape of your body but should not restrict movement. (And if you're feeling adventurous, do a little naked yoga. Seeing yourself in the buff will help you connect and get comfortable with your body. But use some discretion; you don't want to startle anybody!)

Setting Up Your Ashram

Essentially, you can practice yoga anywhere; just make sure the area you choose meets the following criteria:

* The space is big enough that you have plenty of room to move without feeling cramped.

* It has a firm but soft surface to stand on. Carpet is fine; a small rug or a yoga mat will also work well.

* The space is warm. If there's not enough heat in the room (or outside), your muscles will have a tendency to tighten up.

* Make sure the area is free of clutter and anything else you might trip over or that could interfere with your yoga session.

* Although this isn't totally necessary, a quiet, tranquil space will help keep you from being distracted.

Breath Control

Pranayama, or breath control, is an important component of a well-rounded yoga practice. *Prana* isn't actually considered breath; it's said to be a ubiquitous energy or life force (the Chinese call it *chi*) that constantly flows around us and moves through us by way of our breath. By controlling our breath, we are regulating the *prana* that moves in and out of our body. The more *prana* we bring into the body, the more energy and life we ingest, and the better we feel. And that's where the *pranayama* exercises come into play (there is one included at the end of each chapter). They teach us how to breathe better, thus teaching us how to pull in more *prana*. If you find this concept a little too abstract, then just think of the breathing exercises as a way to connect your mind and your body, build lung strength and capacity, and flood your system with energy and vitality. Either way, you win.

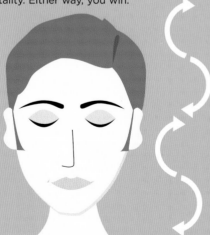

Remember, yoga is a gradual process—a journey, not a competition. Accept your fitness level (both mental and physical) and where your body is willing to go from day to day.

Posture Pointers

* Make sure you practice on an empty stomach. A full belly is uncomfortable, will disrupt your yoga flow, and may make you feel sick.

* Yoga should not be painful. So if something hurts, stop doing it.

* During postures (and most breathing exercises), always breathe through your nose. Generally speaking, inhale during backbends and when limbs extend outward or upward, and exhale during forward bends and when the body is twisting.

* If you're just starting a yoga practice, hold each posture for about three to five full breaths (one full breath equaling an inhalation and an exhalation). As you progress, gradually start holding the postures longer.

* Don't rush. Gently, gracefully flow through each posture. Think grace. Think poise. Think fluidity.

* Yoga is about the here and now, so focus all your attention on each posture. Be aware of yourself and aware of your body.

* Take a few minutes during each session to squeeze in a breathing exercise. This is an important part of your practice and will help build lung strength and bring your mind and body together.

* At the end of your practice, be sure to give yourself at least five minutes to lie in complete stillness (or what is called the Corpse Pose). This will give your body a chance to relax and soak in the benefits of the yoga.

Warming Up

The warm-up is designed to help you loosen up your neck, shoulders, hips, and spine *before* you start your yoga session. Heating up the body and removing stiffness from the muscles and joints will make moving into the postures safer and easier. Spend a few minutes in this section before you venture into the other chapters. Once you feel warmed up and your body feels loose, you've got the green light to get started.

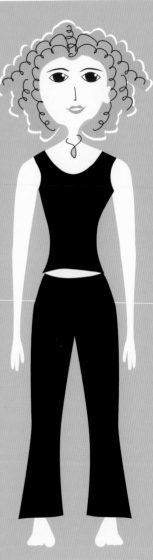

Head Rolls

Sit or stand with a straight back, but allow your neck and shoulder muscles to completely relax.

Slowly and fluidly rotate your head in a full circle to the right and then to the left.

Do five rolls in each direction.

Shoulder Rolls and Squeeze

Stand or kneel and let your hands hang by your sides. Your head, neck, and spine should be straight.

In a continuous circular motion, push your shoulders up and forward and then back and down, bringing your shoulder blades together and expanding your chest.

Continue pushing down, then around and forward again.

Do five to ten rotations.

After your final rotation, put your hands on your waist. Push your chest forward and slowly pull your elbows back and toward one another. Feel the stretch across your chest as your shoulder blades squeeze together.

Continue to squeeze the shoulder blades for a count of ten and release.

Hip Circling

Stand upright with your feet shoulder width apart, your hands on your hips.

Bend your knees slightly, and in an exaggerated but controlled motion, slowly circle your hips to the right, keeping your back straight.

Do fifteen rotations and then switch directions.

Backward and Forward Bend

Stand with your legs hip distance apart. Extend your arms overhead, palms turned in.

Drop your head back and slowly bend backward from the base of your spine. Don't push too hard; remember, you're just warming up.

Take five slow, deep breaths.

Now gently pull yourself up and bend forward. Let your arms and head dangle toward the ground. Relax into the posture. Take five breaths.

Slowly roll yourself up one vertebra at a time and return to center.

Twist

Stand with your feet together and your hands on your hips.

Keeping your hips, legs, and toes facing forward, turn your body to the right and your head to the left, twisting as deeply as you can. Feel the stretch in your neck, shoulders, and spine as you hold the twist for five breaths.

(A deep, soulful groan can sometimes mean the difference between a good stretch and a great stretch, so feel free to vocalize at will.)

Slowly and in control, turn your body to the left and your head to the right, again twisting deeply. Hold for ten to twenty seconds.

Repeat two times.

The Up and Down

Standing with your feet hip distance apart and your knees relaxed, extend your arms out in front of you, palms facing down.

Without using your arms for support, *slowly* sit down on the floor.

Again, without the help of your arms, stand up and return to the starting position.

Repeat ten times.

CHAPTER ONE

Strong Statements

This chapter is designed to help you build a stronger body. While flexibility is an important element of many yoga postures, and is probably what you associate most with the idea of yoga, it's really only one part of your practice. Strength and endurance are also very important components and are the building blocks on which you will base the rest of your practice. The exercises that follow were chosen specifically for their ability to develop strength and stamina. You'll notice that they consist mostly of standing poses; that is intentional. Standing postures are the best and most direct route to a stronger, more powerful you.

Mountain Pose is a proud posture that promotes energy, confidence, and stability. The idea here is simple: Stand up straight. It's easy to get complacent with our posture. Head down, shoulders slouched, we move through life throwing our bodies out of balance and our minds out of focus. But there's an obvious solution to keeping mind and body alert and engaged: Be a mountain, not a molehill.

Mountain Pose

* Look straight ahead. Stand with your feet together, heels and toes touching. Make sure your weight is distributed evenly across the soles of your feet and between your hips and legs.

* Let your arms hang naturally by your sides and lift your chest.

* Contracting your stomach, tilt your hips forward slightly and engage your legs and buttocks.

* Your body should feel strong, but not stiff. Don't overexaggerate any elements of the posture. Your spine should be straight, not arched, and your chin level, not lifted.

* Hold for one minute.

Glow-How

Keep in mind that this is a unique posture, in that you can maintain it to some degree throughout the day. When you find yourself slouching over in your chair or shuffling along with your head down, straighten up and remember: You are a mountain!

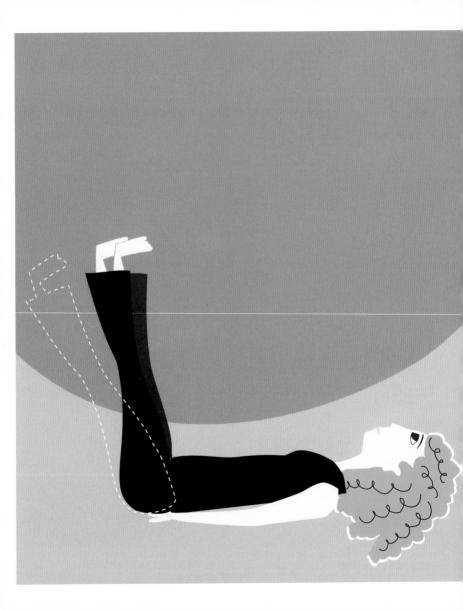

An important component to a strong posture is an engaged stomach. When the stomach muscles are contracted, the lower spine is supported, which leads to a safer, more effective posture. Doing a few leg lifts before breakfast or adding them to your evening exercise regimen will help you build stomach strength and a better all-around yoga practice.

Leg Lifts

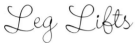

* Lie on your back.

* Tuck your hands, palms down, under your tailbone. Keep your arms straight.

* With your legs engaged and your feet together, inhale and contract your stomach muscles as you gently lift both legs up until they're perpendicular to the floor. Pause for a moment.

* On the exhalation, slowly lower your legs, keeping your feet together and your stomach and legs muscles engaged. Don't let your legs bend or drop; make sure your movements are deliberate and in control. Your stomach muscles might burn a little bit. This is a good thing.

* Do five lifts to start. Once that becomes too easy, try ten.

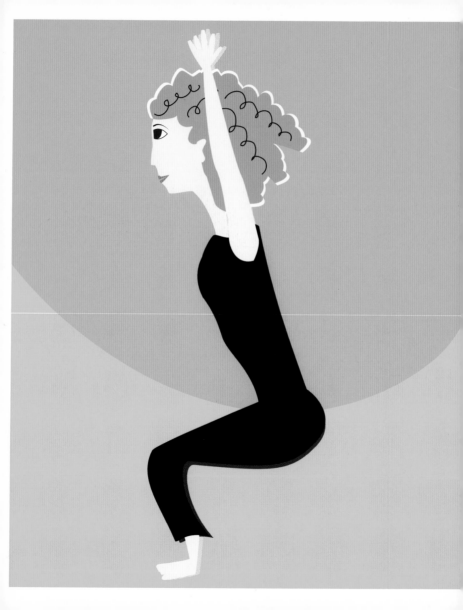

Charge your mind and body with this powerful and dynamic posture. It helps develop chest, back, and leg muscles, build ankle and knee strength, and improve balance. Like lightning, it's quick but concentrated, so do it anywhere—your cubical, a bathroom stall, tucked in a dark corner of the library.

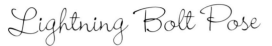

Lightning Bolt Pose

* Stand with your feet and knees together, your arms stretched overhead, palms together.

* Now, as if you were sitting back in a chair, bend your knees and lower your body so that your thighs are parallel to the floor. Make sure your heels don't lift off the ground and your knees don't turn inward.

* Try not to lean forward. Keep your chest lifted and pushed back (you should feel an arch in your spine) and your arms locked and over your ears.

* Hold for three to five breaths and release.

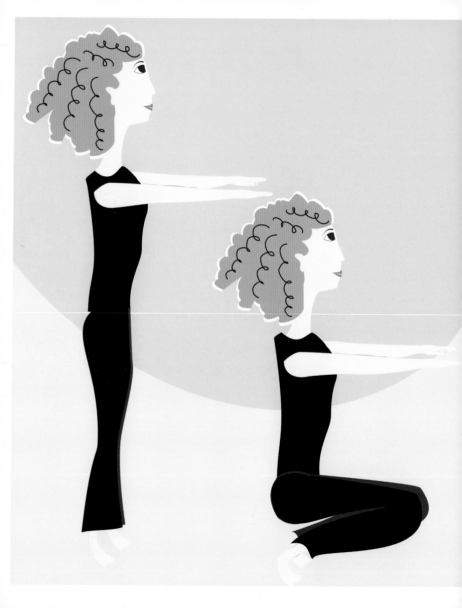

*With strength and stamina come self-confidence and poise.
Developing your body will make you a formidable presence
not only physically but mentally and emotionally as well.
The Toe Squat will help build strength in your feet, ankles,
abdomen, and legs, while toning your arms and back.*

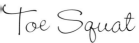

Toe Squat

* Stand with your feet about two fist lengths apart.
  Bring your arms up straight out in front of you, parallel
  to the ground, palms facing down.

* Rise up on your tiptoes, contract your stomach, and
  slowly squat down, keeping your arms and spine straight,
  your chin lifted, and your shoulders pressed down.

* If you can, squat down until your thighs are parallel to
  the floor. Make sure to keep your toes and heels lifted,
  your back straight, and your pelvis tucked under.

* Hold for three to five breaths, then stand up slowly,
  and lower your arms and heels.

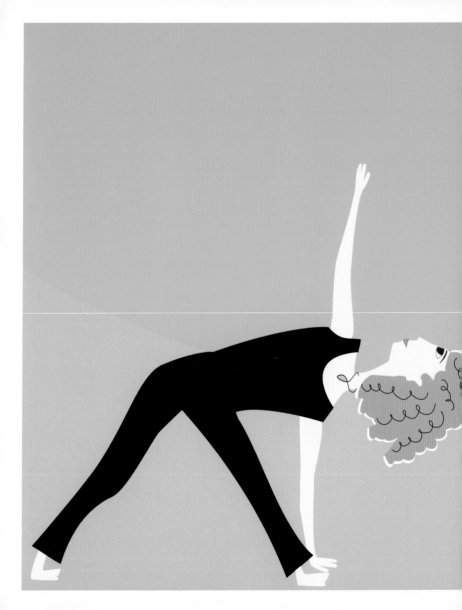

Triangle Pose stretches your chest, arms, and shoulders; tones your back and waist; strengthens your legs and ankles; and stimulates your circulation. It makes for a great stretch after a marathon meeting or any time your muscles need a wake-up call.

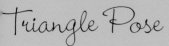

Triangle Pose

* Stand with your feet roughly three to four feet apart. Raise your arms up at your sides so they are level with your shoulders, parallel to the floor, palms facing down.

* Lengthen your neck and spine, and expand your chest. Contract your thighs, point your right foot in slightly, and turn your left foot out about ninety degrees. Rotate your palms forward, turn your chin to your right shoulder, and bend left at your waist, resting your left hand on your left ankle or on the floor behind you.

* Make sure your right arm is perpendicular to the floor and in line with your left arm. Don't collapse into the posture. Your arms, legs, neck, and spine should be straight and engaged, your shoulders in line and pushed back.

* Hold the posture for three to five breaths, then return to center. Repeat on the other side.

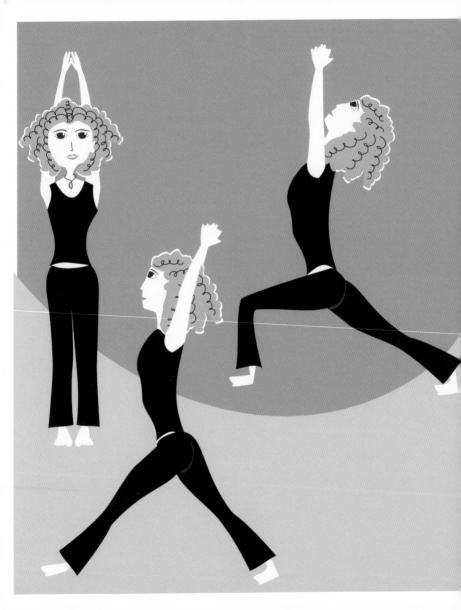

The Warrior Pose is a bold posture that can give you a sense of subtle strength and serene power. More than just an exercise, it awakens your fighting spirit as it strengthens your ankles, knees, legs, and hips, and relieves a stiff neck and tense shoulders. Do a quick Warrior on your lunch break or between classes, and for the rest of the afternoon carry yourself with the confidence and presence of a modern-day heroine.

Warrior I

* Stand straight with your feet together. Raise your arms overhead until they cover your ears. Your elbows should be locked and your palms together.

* Step to the side about four feet. Rotate to the right so that your right foot is pointed forward and your left foot is angled out just slightly.

* Bend your right knee so that your right thigh is parallel with the floor. Your ankle and knee should be in line, perpendicular to the floor. Your hips should be square, and your left leg should be straight and solid, foot planted, heel on the floor.

* Drop your head back and look up at your hands. Hold the pose for three to five breaths, then return to center. Repeat on the other side.

Glow-How

If you're looking for a slightly easier version of Warrior, try Warrior II. Begin as you do in Warrior I, but this time raise your arms so they are parallel to the ground, look to the right, and bend your right leg, keeping your upper body erect and facing forward. Repeat on the other side.

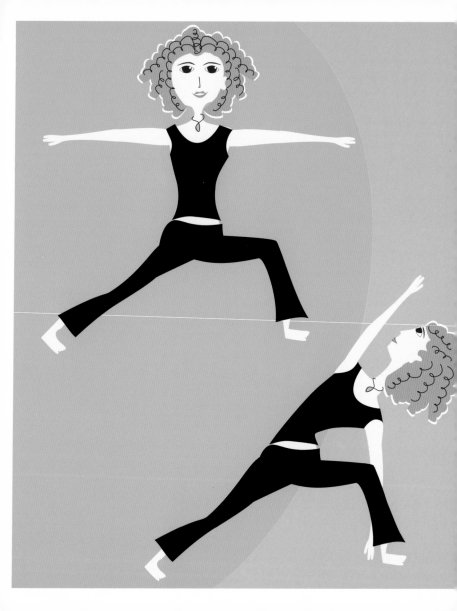

Yoga helps you reestablish a more intimate relationship with your body, showing you the areas with strength and flexibility as well as other areas that may need some extra love and attention. Extended-Angle Pose is a great way to reconnect with your muscles, joints, and organs. It not only opens up the heart, flooding your veins with energy and vitality, but also stretches and strengthens virtually every muscle group in the body.

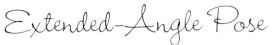

Extended-Angle Pose

Glow-How

During the more challenging postures, your muscles may shake and quiver a bit at first. Don't worry: As you get stronger, the shaking will subside.

* Stand with your feet about four feet apart. Turn your right foot out ninety degrees and turn your left foot in slightly.

* Raise your arms up so they are shoulder height and parallel to the floor, palms down.

* Lunge to the right, bending your right knee so that your leg forms a right angle with the floor—the knee directly over the ankle, the thigh parallel to the floor, the shin perpendicular. Keep your left leg straight and engaged.

* Turn your head to the left and, in a controlled motion, bend your upper body to the right.

* Rest your right palm on the floor behind your foot as you extend your left arm over your head so that it forms a straight line from your fingertips to your left ankle.

* Your chest, hips, and legs should be aligned and your whole body should be engaged.

* Hold the pose for three to five breaths, then repeat on the other side.

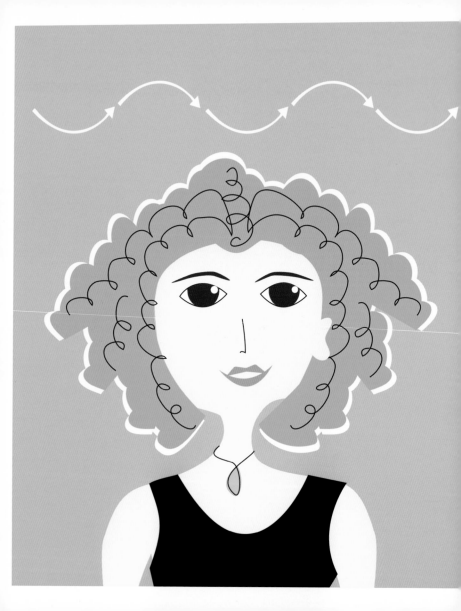

Breathing is instinctual, but breathing well is not. For most of us, bad breathing habits run so deep that we don't even notice we're breathing at all. Holding your breath is a simple technique that will help you learn breath control. This may seem like kid stuff, but it's a great way to get to know your lungs and increase your lung strength and capacity.

Hold It!

* Sit comfortably and take a deep breath through your nose. Your lungs should feel full, but not to the point of discomfort.

* Relax and hold the breath for as long as you can. Make sure you remain comfortable and calm. No passing out and no turning blue!

* Exhale steadily through your nose. If the air bursts loudly from the mouth or nose on the exhalation, you've held your breath for too long. No need to go for the world record here—just hold it until your body tells you it's time to come up for air.

* Repeat two times.

CHAPTER TWO

Blissful Balancers

In this chapter, not only will you learn to balance your right side with your left side and your front side with your back side, but you will also learn the delicate balance of mind and body. Concentration is just as important to achieving balance as coordination. In fact, it's the two together that make for a successful posture.

Learning how to balance can be a challenge and will take practice and patience. There will most certainly be days when you're feeling off-kilter, or your mind is scattered, and you'll wobble and probably topple over. Don't get discouraged; it's all part of the process. The more you practice, the more your mind and body will learn to work together, and the easier balancing will become.

Focus on the rhythm inherent in this posture. It will help calm your soul, clear your head, and center your mind.

Leg Pendulum

* Stand straight with your feet together, your hands resting on your hips.

* Shift your weight onto your right leg, engaging your right thigh muscles.

* Keeping your body balanced and centered, swing your left leg forward and backward from the hip in a controlled motion. Make sure your body remains upright and engaged and your left leg is relaxed and straight.

* Continue swinging your leg for five full breaths, then repeat on the other side.

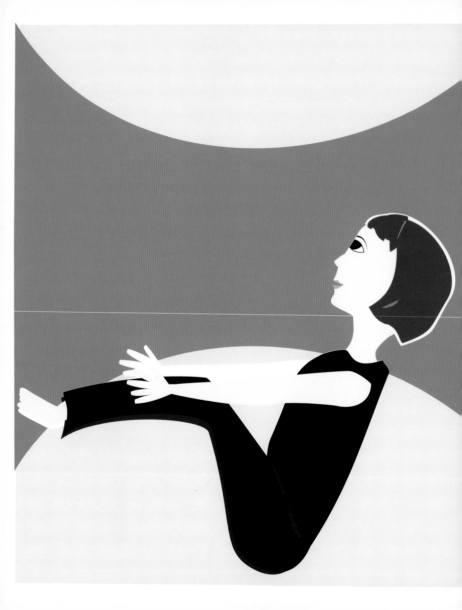

This posture gives you the opportunity to fine-tune your focus and balance while also strengthening your stomach and back muscles and toning your arms. If you capsize at first, not to worry; it's only a matter of time until you'll have the stamina and balance to keep this pose afloat.

Half Boat Pose

* Sit on the floor with your knees bent.

* Slowly and simultaneously lean back and bring your feet off the floor. Balance on your buttocks. Extend your arms out so they are next to your legs and parallel to the floor. Turn your palms in.

* Keeping your knees bent and together, raise your feet so that your lower legs are parallel to the floor.

* Hold for three to five breaths and release.

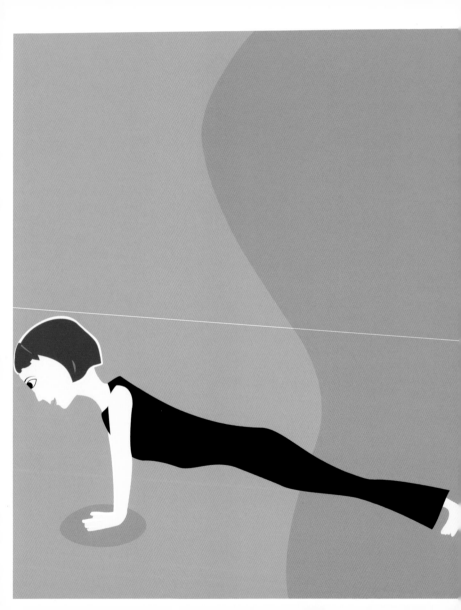

This is a strong and steady pose. It improves posture and builds muscle strength in the arms, shoulders, back, legs, and feet. Use it to ground your energy and center your mind and body.

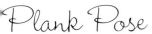

Plank Pose

* Lie down on your stomach. Place your hands directly under your shoulders, palms down, fingers forward.

* Tuck your toes under so the soles of your feet are perpendicular to the floor.

* Push up, straightening your arms. Your body should be supported entirely by your palms and toes.

* Make sure your body is completely straight from your head to your ankles—no sagging legs or arching back.

* Hold for three to five breaths, then slowly lower your body back down to the ground.

Glow-How

Remember, put as much effort and energy into your yoga practice as you have to give. If you're over-loaded with work or are catching a late-night movie, maybe squeeze in a posture or two before bed. If you're enjoying the evening solo, spend a half hour on your yoga practice. Assess your weaker areas and choose your postures accordingly. Is your back tight? Focus on the forward and backward bends. Do you need to relax? Try a breathing exercise.

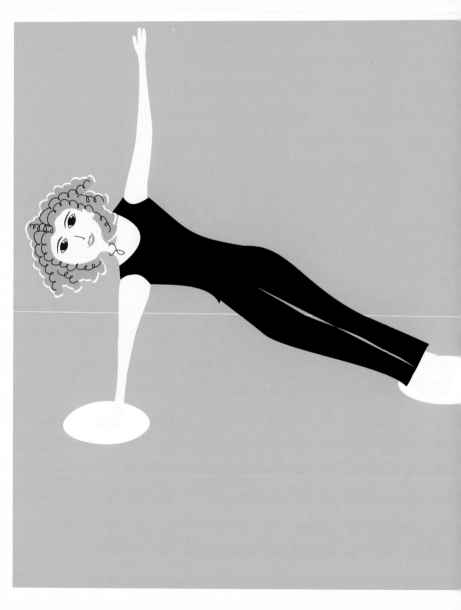

This posture develops balance and concentration, strengthens the wrists and arms, and tones the lower back. Be forewarned: You may feel the urge to yell out, "Hey, look what I can do!" And that's okay. Taking pride in yourself and in your practice is encouraged.

Side Inclined Plane

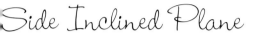

* Get in the push-up position (also known as the Plank Pose), with your hands directly under your shoulders, arms and legs straight.

* Turn your body to the right without bending your arms, legs, or back.

* Stack your feet one on top of the other, and lift your right arm straight up in the air, palm facing forward. Your body should be in a straight line, diagonal to the floor, and the entire front side of your body should be facing forward.

* Keep your body engaged and straight. Don't let your hips sag toward the floor; that will put unnecessary stress on your back and arm.

* Hold for three breaths, release, and switch sides.

A quick knee squeeze will stretch your legs and hips and help build a balanced body and a steady mind. Try doing this posture mindfully. How does your body feel? Where are your muscles tense? Be present with yourself and focus on your body.

Standing Knee Squeeze

* Stand up straight with your feet together and your arms hanging by your sides.

* Shift your weight onto your right leg, engaging the thigh muscle.

* Lift your left knee up as far as you can without throwing yourself off balance.

* Grab your left leg about an inch below the knee with interlocked fingers.

* Keeping your chin level, look straight ahead, lengthen your body up, and pull your knee to your body. Keep your torso straight, your hips square, and your shoulders relaxed and down.

* Breathe naturally and hold for three to five breaths.

* Repeat on the other side.

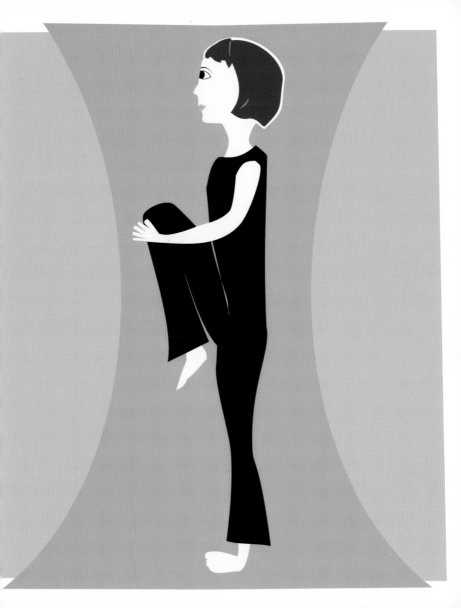

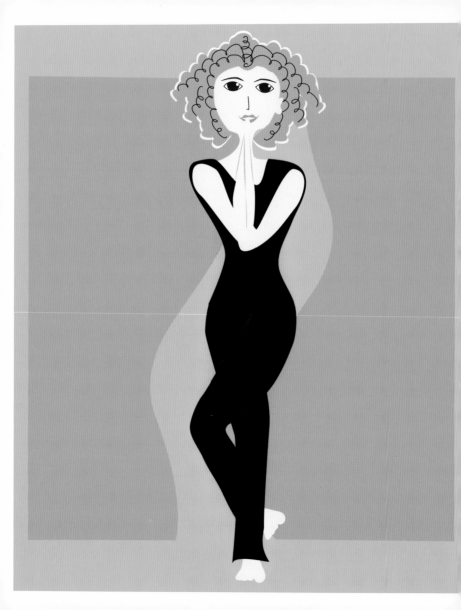

The Eagle pose is one of the tougher balancing postures, but don't be intimidated. Part of yoga is believing in yourself and having confidence in your mind and body. The key: Stay focused and breathe into it. Not only will you see improved balance, but this exercise will also develop leg and ankle strength, tone the back and abdomen, and stretch all twelve major joints of the body.

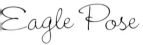

Eagle Pose

* Begin with your feet together, spine straight, chest lifted, knees slightly bent, hands at your sides.

* Bend your elbows and swing your right arm underneath your left. Wrap your forearms so that your palms meet in front of your face— they should be in the prayer position. Try to keep your fingertips level and below your nose.

* Bend your knees, crouching down as low as you can. Lift your right leg up and over your left leg, crossing your thighs, and hook your right foot around your left ankle.

* With your chest lifted, hips level, and stomach sucked in, try to line up your wrist, knee, and ankle joints in a row down the front of your body. Balance there for three breaths.

Glow-How

Feeling a little funny? That's okay. This one may take some practice, but stick with it—your body and mind will thank you.

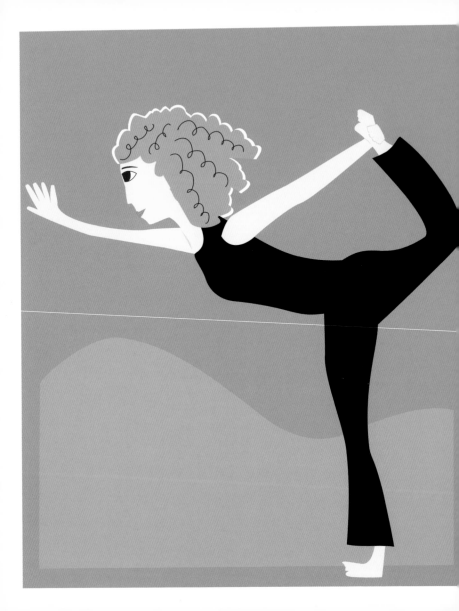

As its name denotes, this is a graceful and beautiful posture. It brings out the hidden prima ballerina in us all as it strengthens and stretches the legs, improves the balance, and tones the back and spine.

Dancing Shiva

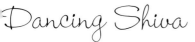

* Standing straight, extend your left arm straight over your head, bend your right knee behind your body, and grasp your right foot from the inside with your right hand.

* Make sure your left arm is next to your ear, palm facing forward, and your left leg is straight and engaged.

* Stretch your left arm forward as you slowly tilt your body down until your left arm and torso are parallel to the ground. Keep your left leg straight and engaged, your hips level, and your chin lifted.

* Slowly, gently kick your right leg into your hand. If you're having a hard time balancing, you may not be kicking enough.

* Hold for three to five breaths, release, and switch sides.

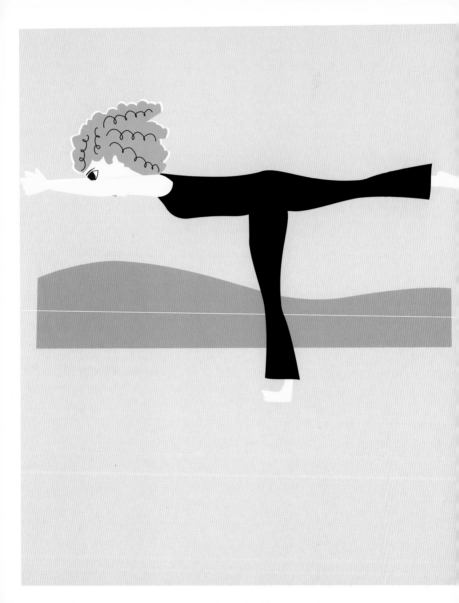

You'll feel like a seasoned yoga veteran once you've conquered this posture. It's one of the more difficult balancing poses, but it is well worth the battle. A few moments in Warrior III will strengthen your arms, legs, and abdomen; tone your hips, chest, back, and neck; stretch your hamstrings; and improve your balance and concentration. Charge!

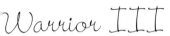

Warrior III

* Stand straight with your feet together.

* Step to the side about four feet. Rotate to the right so that your right foot is pointed forward and your left foot is angled out just slightly. Raise arms so they are parallel to the ground, palms down.

* Bend your right knee so that your right thigh is parallel with the floor. Your ankle and knee should be in line, perpendicular to the floor. Your left leg should be straight and solid, your left foot planted.

* Lean forward over your right thigh as you slowly straighten your right leg and lift your left leg. Raise your arms overhead so that they cover your ears. Your elbows should be locked and your palms together.

* Continue bending forward until your arms, torso, and left leg are parallel to the floor and your right leg is perpendicular to the floor, resembling a T. Make sure your hips are level, your chin is forward, and your legs and arms remain straight and engaged.

* Hold for three to five breaths, return to center, and repeat on the other side.

This breathing exercise balances your physical and emotional energies. When you're feeling off-kilter, it's a great way to calm your mind, relax your body, and come back to center.

Alternate-Nostril Breathing

* Sit comfortably in a chair or cross-legged on the floor. Make sure your back and neck are straight and your shoulders are relaxed.

* Rest your left hand, palm up, in your lap or on your left thigh. Fold the middle and index fingers of your right hand over so they touch your palm.

* Bring your right hand up to your nose. Close your eyes. Gently close your right nostril with your thumb and exhale through your left nostril.

* When your lungs are empty, take a deep, steady inhalation through your left nostril. Make sure your facial muscles remain relaxed.

* Close your left nostril with the ring and pinkie fingers so that both nostrils are sealed. Hold there for a few seconds.

* Open your right nostril only and exhale slowly and steadily. When the air is completely emptied, pause for a moment, then inhale through your right nostril until your lungs are full.

* Close your right nostril. Again, both nostrils are blocked. Hold for a moment.

* Release your left nostril and expel the air. When your lungs are empty, take a deep breath through your left nostril. This completes one breathing cycle.

* Repeat three times.

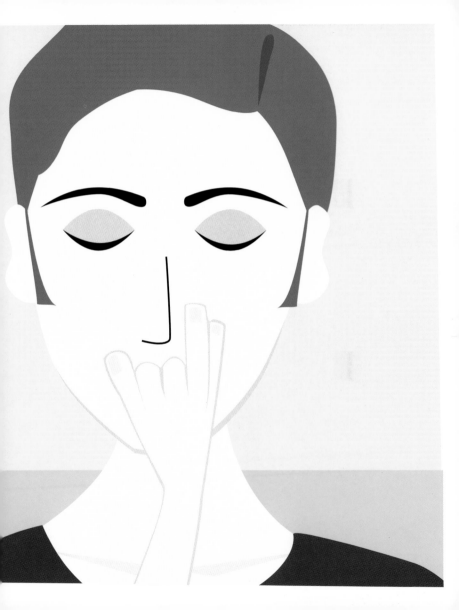

CHAPTER THREE

Essential Energizers

The goal of this chapter is simple: to flood your body with energy and vitality. Yoga in general will help revitalize you, but the postures that follow were selected in particular for their keen ability to energize the body and stimulate the mind. Backbends, twists, and inversions all have the capacity to invigorate you, so at least one of each has been included in this chapter. They all have their own subtle way of enlivening your system, so give each one a try and see what works best for you. There are a few postures stuck in between the backbends that aren't necessarily powerful energizers; they are there simply to act as counterstretches to the intense back compressions, should you choose to do the entire chapter in sequence.

Cobra is the perfect posture when you need a quick pick-me-up. Like all backbends, it energizes the body and stimulates the brain and circulatory system. It also helps to align and strengthen the spine.

Cobra Pose

* Lie facedown on the floor with your feet together and your toes pointed. Place your hand on either side of your chest, palms down, elbows tucked into your body. Tighten your legs and buttocks. (Remember to maintain this locked cobra tail throughout the posture.)

* Inhale while slowly, in succession, raising your head, chin, neck, shoulders, and chest by contracting your back muscles. Keep your shoulders down, your face relaxed, and press your hips, legs, and feet against the floor. Lift as high as you can.

* This is a back-strengthening exercise, so don't use your arms to push your body up—that's cheating! Rely on your back muscles when lifting.

* Look up, hold the pose for three to five breaths, and slowly roll down.

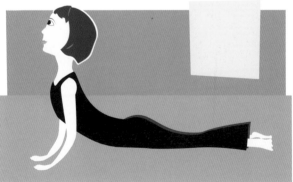

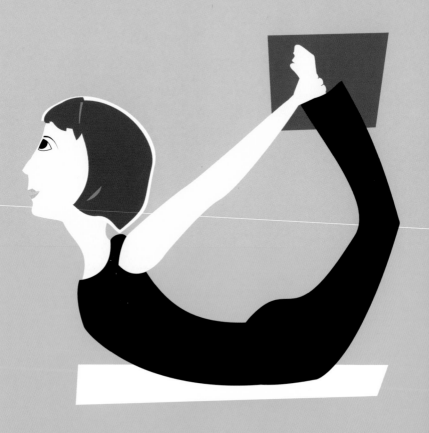

Bow pose is a tremendously invigorating posture that will leave you feeling refreshed, renewed, and free of tense muscles and tired thoughts. As it stretches and lengthens the front side of the body, it compresses the entire spine, stimulating circulation and strengthening the back muscles. Ahhh!

Bow Pose

* Lie on your stomach.

* Bend your knees and reach back with your arms, grabbing the outside of the right ankle with the right arm and the outside of the left ankle with the left arm. Make sure you have a firm grip.

* Lift your legs and chest simultaneously and pull your arms taut (like the string of a bow). Feel the front of your body lengthening as your buttocks and spine compress.

* Keep your arms straight and your shoulders pressed down.

* Tilt your head back, relax your face, and look up.

* Hold for three to five breaths and release.

Glow-How

Yoga should not be painful. That doesn't mean, however, that it's okay to wimp out. You'll see and feel the best results if you push yourself; go to your edge and linger there for a few breaths before releasing.

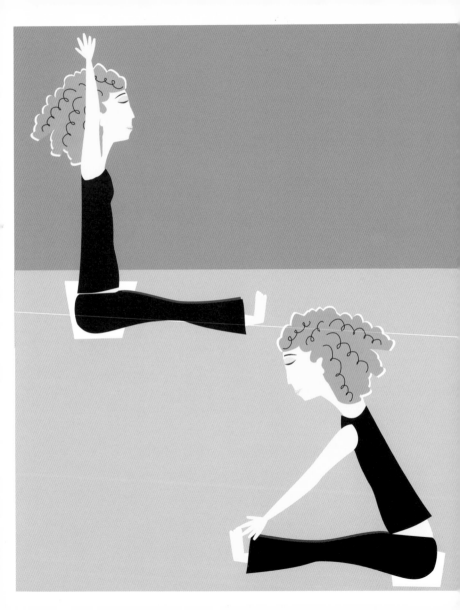

This seemingly simple posture rejuvenates the entire spine while stretching the back side of the body from head to toe.

Sitting Forward Bend

* Sit on the floor with your legs together and extended straight out in front of you.

* Lift your arms above your head, lean forward from your hips, and grab your toes. Wrap the first two fingers and thumb of your right hand around your right big toe and the first two fingers and thumb of your left hand around your left big toe.

* Extending from the hips, push your torso forward toward your legs. Try to keep your back flat and your legs straight.

* Using your arms as levers, pull your body forward. Feel your spine lengthening.

* Hold for three to five breaths and release.

There's nothing like a good spinal twist to wring out stress, tension, and anything else that may be polluting the mind and body. As it stretches and aligns your spine, it stimulates your internal organs, helping the body free itself of any lingering toxins in the tissues.

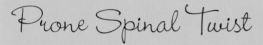

Prone Spinal Twist

* Lie down on your back and extend your arms out from your shoulders, perpendicular to your body.

* Bring your knees up to your chest and then let them drop to your right side as you turn your head to the left. Try to keep both shoulders on the ground.

* Relax and hold the pose for three to five breaths.

* Bring your knees and head back to center and repeat on the other side.

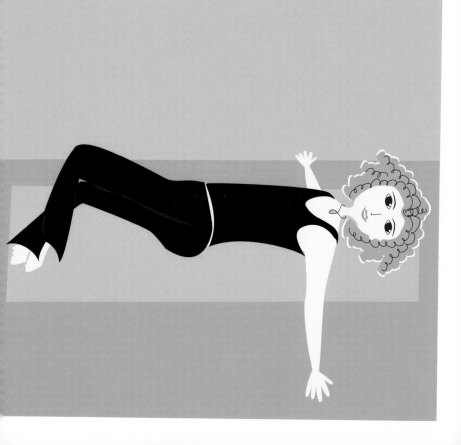

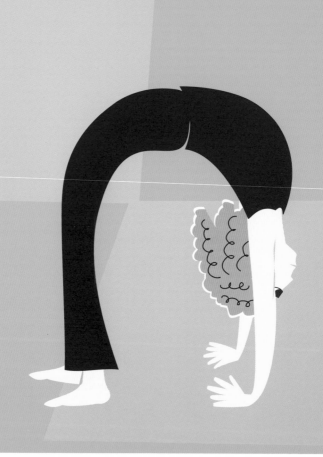

For those of you who did backyard gymnastics as a kid, this is your basic backbend. Believe it or not, our old childhood favorite is one of the most powerful yoga postures. It stretches the belly; tones the legs, buttocks, and arms; increases energy; and improves circulation and concentration. If you're having a memory lapse, just follow the instructions below.

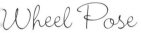

Wheel Pose

* Lie on your back with knees bent, feet flat on the floor, heels tucked up against the buttocks.

* Bring your palms to the floor next to your head, fingers facing your feet, elbows bent.

* Raise your torso up and rest the top of your head on the ground.

* Push up again, lifting your belly toward the sky, arching your back. Your body should resemble an archway, arms and legs approaching straight, head lifted off the floor.

* Hold for five breaths and slowly come down.

Glow-How

If the full posture is a little bit too challenging for you, not to worry—you can work your way up to it. To start, try keeping your arms and legs bent slightly. If that's still too much, gently rest your head on the floor between your hands.

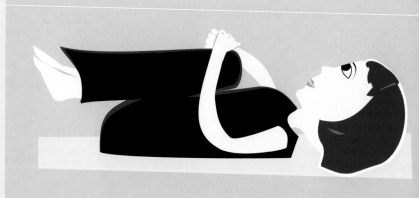

This posture relaxes the lower back and stretches the hips and legs. It isn't meant to jolt your system with energy like the other poses in the chapter; rather, its purpose is to act as a counterpose to the Wheel Pose. Use it after any of the back-bends included in this book, and keep it in mind if you decide to create your own yoga sequence.

Knees-to-Chest Pose

* Lie on your back and bring your knees up to your chest with your feet together and your chin on your chest.

* Wrap your arms around your knees, gripping your wrists, forearms, or elbows.

* Pull your knees toward your chest as your push your pelvis down toward the floor, flattening out your back.

* Hold for three to five breaths and release.

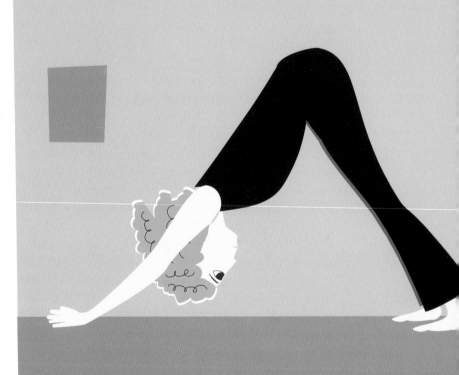

Downward Dog is a quick and easy posture that increases energy and removes stiffness in the legs, back, and shoulders. You'll be as loose and spirited as a puppy after a few moments in this posture.

Downward-Facing Dog

* Start from a standing position. Bend over, place your hands firmly on the ground (about shoulder width apart), and take a few steps back. Adjust your feet so that they are hip width apart. Your body should resemble an inverted V.

* Press your hands and heels flat to the floor as you lift your tailbone toward the ceiling, tightening your legs and abdomen, and lengthening your lower back.

* Make sure that your back is straight, not curved, and that your arms are fully extended (i.e., no bend in the elbow) and your neck relaxed.

* Hold for three to five breaths. Walk your feet up to your hands, roll up into the starting position, and repeat.

Glow-How

Water is vital to a healthy and happy mind and body. When we don't have a sufficient amount (at least eight glasses a day), our energy level suffers. Here are a few tips on how to stay hydrated and keep your energy flowing:

* Have a glass of water when you wake up in the morning.

* Always have a cup (or bottle) of water within reach during the day.

* Make a habit of drinking water instead of coffee or that sugar-laden, carbonated stuff.

* Whenever you pass the water cooler, stop and have a sip.

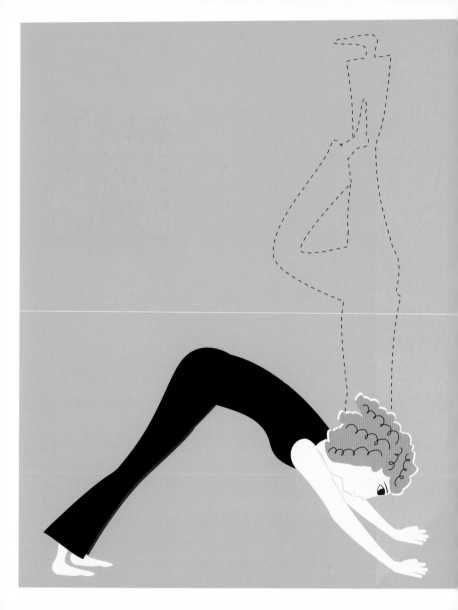

The handstand pumps your body with energy while it strengthens your arms, shoulders, wrists, and abdomen— oh, and it's a lot of fun. If you're a little intimidated, ask a friend to give you a hand.

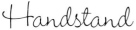

Handstand

* Stand in front of a wall. Bend forward and place your hands about five inches from the wall, shoulder width apart. Your feet should be about three feet behind your hands.

* Walk your legs closer to the wall. Push off with your left leg as you lift your right leg straight up, followed immediately by your left leg. Rest them both against the wall. Keep your arms and legs straight and engaged and your stomach tightened.

* Hold for three to five breaths, then carefully drop your legs to the ground.

This simple breathing exercise was named after the proud chest often associated with the victorious and triumphant. It is an invigorating and energizing form of deep breathing that calms the mind, oxygenates the blood, and tones the nervous and respiratory systems. Give it a try before your next conquest.

#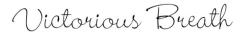

- Sit up straight with your hands resting in your lap or relaxed on your thighs.

- Exhale all of the air from your lungs. Contracting your throat muscles slightly, inhale a slow, even, continuous flow of air through your nose. If you hear a low hissing sound as you breathe in, you're doing it right. If not, try again.

- Continue to inhale until your lungs are comfortably full. Feel your chest expand and rise slightly.

- Hold this breath for a few seconds. Now, in the same fashion as your inhalation, exhale slowly, evenly, and continuously. Again, making the hissing sound.

- Take ten full breaths. (An inhalation and an exhalation is considered one full breath.)

CHAPTER FOUR

Meltdown Menders

The postures and exercises in this chapter are meant to help you calm down, relax, and let go. Take it slow. Allow yourself the time to take care of your mind and your body. Ease into the postures. Feel stress, tension, and anxiety float away as you go deeper and deeper into each stretch, and deeper and deeper into a state of peace and serenity. Take this opportunity to empty your mind. Don't think, don't worry, don't analyze. The world around you should cease to exist. In this chapter, it's just you, your body, and your breath.

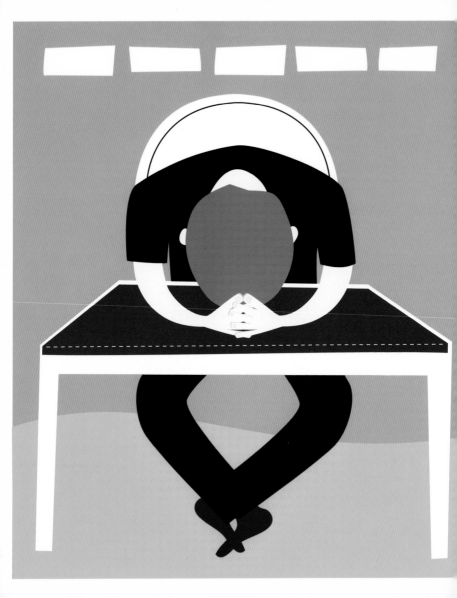

Never ignore cries for attention from your mind or body. There's always time to take a moment to relax and regroup. Next time you're weary with stress and tension, try this simple exercise. It will calm your body and settle your mind.

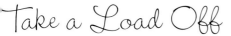

Take a Load Off

* Sit in a chair in front of your desk or at a table. Make sure you are close enough to the table that when you bend forward, your forehead can rest comfortably on it.

* Gently place your forehead on the table and fold your arms around your head.

* Relax and breathe normally. Let go of any tension in your neck, shoulders, and spine.

* Hold the position for three to five breaths.

Use this posture as a chance to let go. Let go of tension in your body, let go of negative thoughts and pent-up emotions, let go of time constraints and commitments, and just hang loose and enjoy.

Hang Loose

* Standing with your back against a wall, bring your heels together and point your toes out slightly.

* One vertebra at a time, slowly roll your body forward until your hands are dangling just below your knees.

* Let go of any tension, and let your head, neck, and arms totally relax.

* Swing your hands in slow and steady circles, first in an inward motion, then in an outward motion.

* Hold the pose for three to five breaths and slowly roll your body up, again, vertebra by vertebra.

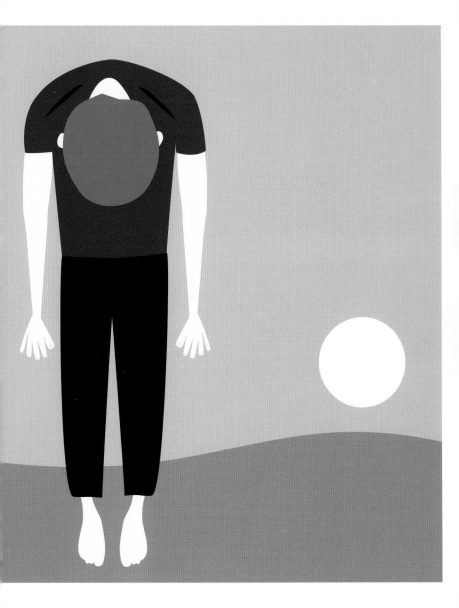

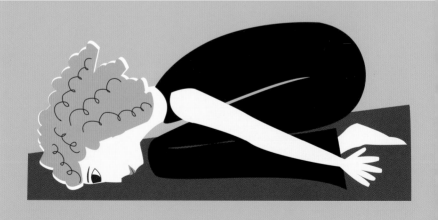

Don't worry if something cataclysmic happens at work or school and your only inclination is to curl up in the fetal position. It's the perfect thing to do. The Child Pose is a comforting and nurturing posture that rests the body and calms the nervous system. A few minutes of this and you'll be reborn.

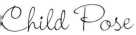

Child Pose

* Kneel on the ground with your knees and feet together. Sit back on your heels.

* Let your arms hang by your sides with the backs of your hands and your fingers resting on the floor by your feet.

* Slowly lower your forehead to the floor, folding your body forward and rounding your back.

* Breathe deeply and steadily. Let your entire body relax.

* Hold for three to five breaths.

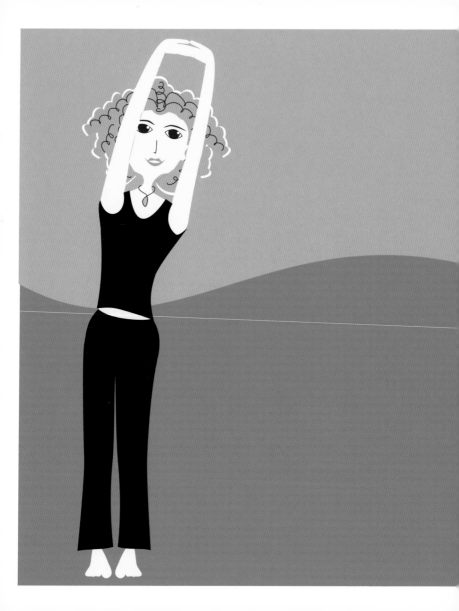

Many of us accumulate tension throughout the day and carry it into the night, where it haunts our sleep. Yoga is a great way to slow down your mind, relax your body, and prepare your soul for slumber. This posture an excellent full-body stretch and is the perfect precursor to a good night's sleep.

Upstretched Arms Pose

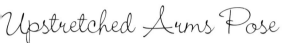

* Stand with your feet together, your spine and neck straight.

* Bring your arms up and over your head, interlocking all ten fingers and turning your palms toward the ceiling. Your arms should be straight and engaged.

* Pull your arms back behind your ears and up from your shoulders, stretching and lengthening your entire body.

* Maintaining this straight stance, push your hips to the left and bend to the right. Make sure your chin stays up, your arms are straight, and your stomach is engaged.

* Hold for three to five breaths, bring yourself back to center, and repeat on the other side.

Glow-How

More Tips for a Better Night's Sleep:

* Take a hot bath.

* Do an evening meditation.

* Try a breathing exercise.

* Enlist your partner for a massage.

* Have a cup of chamomile tea.

* Spray a mist of lavender oil and water on your pillow.

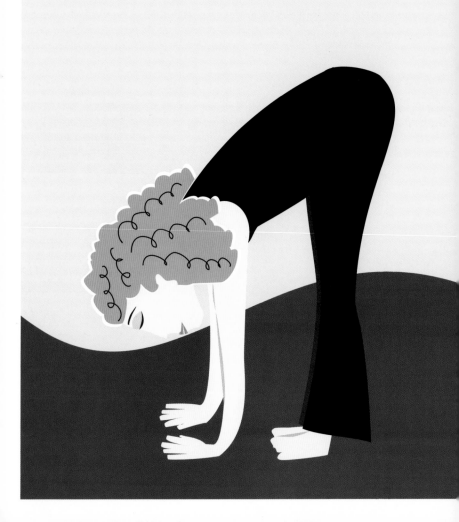

Experiencing a system overload? Before you spontaneously combust, try this simple posture. It will settle your nervous system and release tense back muscles and tight hamstrings to help you let go and really relax.

Standing Forward Bend

* Stand up straight with your feet together.

* Extend your arms overhead and slowly bend forward from the hips, placing your hands in front of your feet or on the backs of your ankles.

* Push your heels into the ground while lifting your hips toward the ceiling.

* Breathe into the stretch. Feel your hamstrings release and your spine lengthen.

* Hold for three to five breaths and slowly roll your body up.

Glow-How

If you are creating your own yoga sequence, this is a great posture to use as a resting position between other standing poses.

Cobbler Pose is a peaceful posture that helps relieve anxiety, improve circulation, and stretch the knees, inner thighs, and groin. Steal a moment between meetings or classes and mend your tired mind and body.

Cobbler Pose

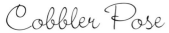

Glow-How

If you're looking to add a back-stretch to this posture, simply fold your upper body over your bent legs. Don't overexert yourself. Let your body ease down slowly and gently.

* Sit with your legs extended out in front of you.

* Bend both legs, place the soles of your feet together, and drop your knees down toward the floor.

* Pull your heels in as close to your pelvis as you can without discomfort and push them together. Grasp the big toe of each foot with the first two fingers and thumb of each corresponding hand.

* Sit up straight with your pelvis in a neutral position and your shoulders relaxed and down.

* Hold for at least five breaths, then release.

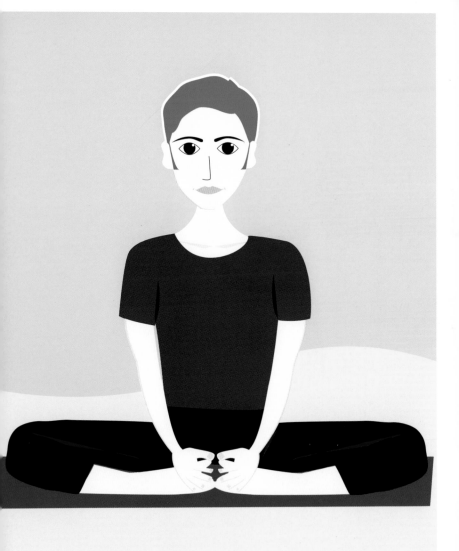

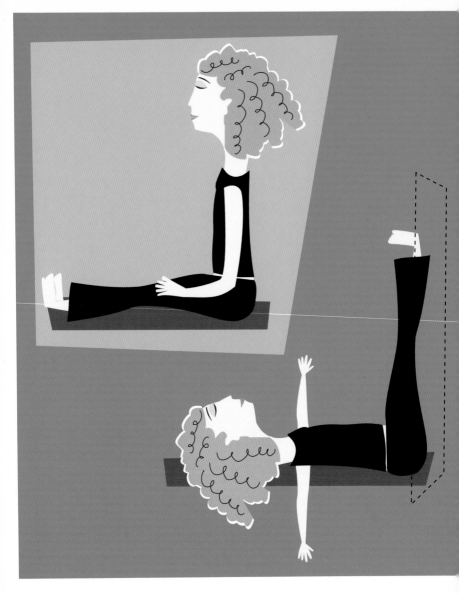

Give those dogs a rest! This exercise will relax and revitalize your entire body, so don't rush it. Give yourself a few minutes and really let go. Feel your body releasing the day's tension as your mind purges unnecessary thoughts and emotions.

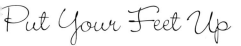

Put Your Feet Up

* Sit down beside a wall, your legs out in front of you.

* Lie back on the floor and slide your legs up on the wall.

* Once your legs are straight and stable, scoot your buttocks up against the wall.

* Stretch your arms out parallel with the wall, palms down.

* Relax every muscle, joint, and organ. Breathe deeply.

* Lie here for at least five minutes, more if you have the time.

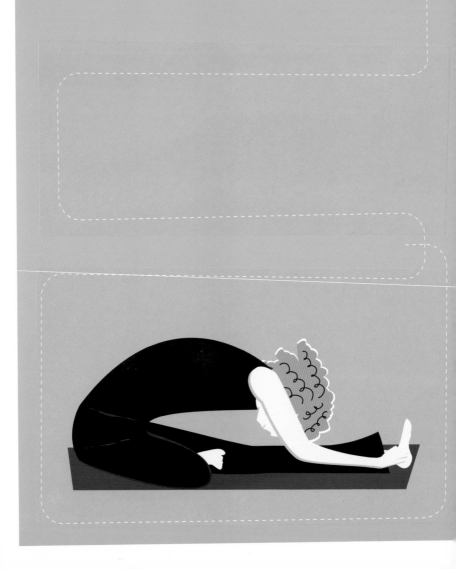

Slow down with this gentle seated posture. It will help settle a frazzled mind as it stretches the back and hamstrings, strengthens the chest, and tones the abdomen.

Sitting Head-to-Knee Pose

* Sit on the floor with both legs extended out in front of you.

* Bend your left leg in and place the sole of your left foot against the inside of your right thigh.

* Clasp your hands and raise them over your head, lengthening your torso.

* Bend forward over your right leg, placing your clasped hands around your right foot and bringing your head to your knee. (If you need to bend the right leg slightly to do this, that's fine.)

* Hold for three to five breaths, lift up to center, and repeat on the other side.

This pranayama *breathing exercise settles the nervous system, calming the mind and body. When you're in need of some peace and tranquility, find a quiet spot and breathe.*

Breath Extension and Retention

* Breathe naturally. Slowly pull yourself into the present moment—present with yourself and present with your breath. Notice the pattern of your breath. Are your breaths deep and steady or quick and shallow? How is your body responding to your breath?

* Start breathing in slowly, deeply, continuously, until your lungs are full. Hold your breath for a moment and then breathe out, slowly and evenly.

* As you settle into your breathing, begin to make your exhalation longer than your inhalation.

* Start with breathing in for three counts, holding your breath for a few seconds, and then breathing out for six counts.

* Eventually you'll want to hold your breath for the same length of time as your exhalation, so you'll breathe in for three, hold for six, and breathe out for six.

CHAPTER FIVE

Blues Busters

Yoga can be very effective therapy. Moving your body, focusing your mind, and stabilizing your breath often have a tonic effect on your mood. This chapter is filled with a combination of postures that will give you a mental and physical lift when, for whatever reason, you're feeling a little low. Be gentle with yourself and don't fight your emotions. As you stretch, acknowledge your feelings, sit with them for a moment, and then let them go.

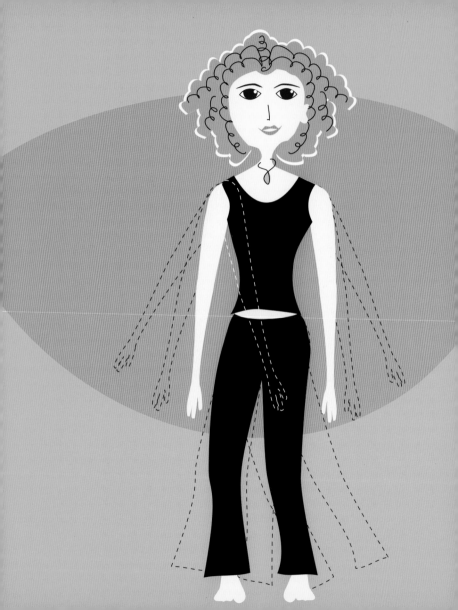

Sometimes life isn't fair. Shake it off, literally. This exercise will not only banish a blue mood, it will also improve circulation and relax your body.

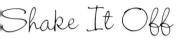

Shake It Off

* Stand straight with your knees slightly bent, your arms at your sides, and your feet hip distance apart.

* Relax your entire body.

* Now vigorously shake out your arms, legs, and torso. Your body should feel loose and free of all tension.

* Let your arms dangle from your shoulders and your hands flop from your wrists.

* Shake until you're exhausted or someone asks if you need a paramedic, whichever comes first.

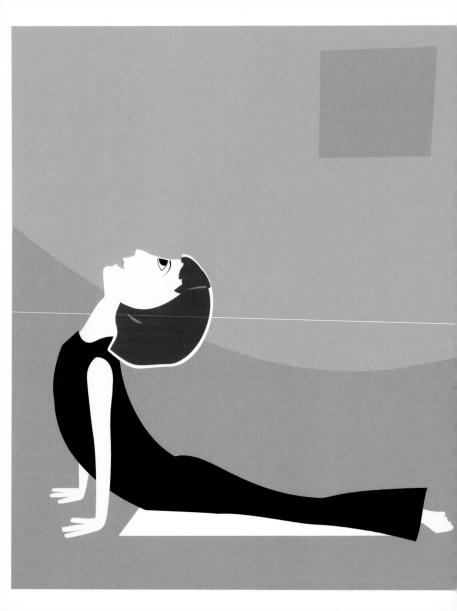

This traditional back-compression posture will invigorate you from head to toe. As it strengthens the spine, it stimulates the nervous system and increases the circulation.

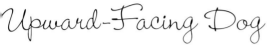

Upward-Facing Dog

* Lie on the floor facedown with your feet together and toes pointed.

* Place your hands on either side of your chest with your palms down, your elbows tucked into your body, and your legs and buttocks contracted.

* Inhale while slowly, in succession, raising your head, chin, neck, shoulders, and chest by contracting your back muscles. Keep your shoulders down and press your hips, legs, and feet together and against the floor.

* Straighten your arms, and in a forward, upward motion, slowly lift the front of your body off the floor. Make sure your legs remain straight and engaged.

* Continue lifting until your hips and legs are slightly off the floor. Look up.

* Hold for three to five breaths and release.

Agility and flexibility are imperative to problem solving. It's not necessarily what happens in life that makes us happy (or unhappy), but rather how we choose to handle it. Let the Cat Pose serve as a reminder of these stellar feline qualities. Just like a cat, you can bounce back. (This posture also stretches the spine, tones the nervous system, and improves the circulation.)

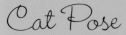

Cat Pose

* Get down on all fours.

* Place your hands directly under your shoulders, arms locked, fingers facing forward.

* Your thighs should be perpendicular to the ground with your knees together and your back flat.

* Lift your chin and head up and arch your back. Hold for three breaths.

* Now lower your head so it is between your arms and push your back up toward the ceiling. Hold for three breaths.

* Rest and repeat.

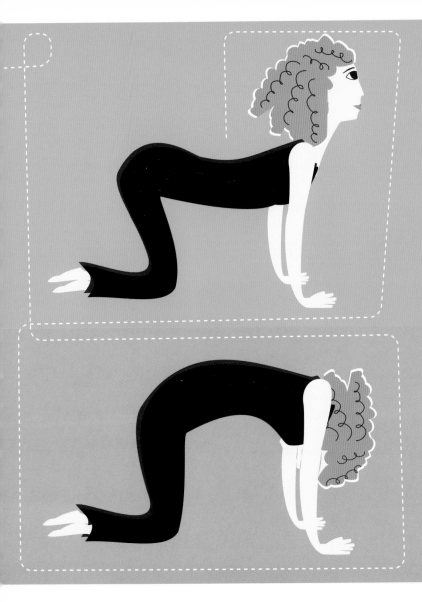

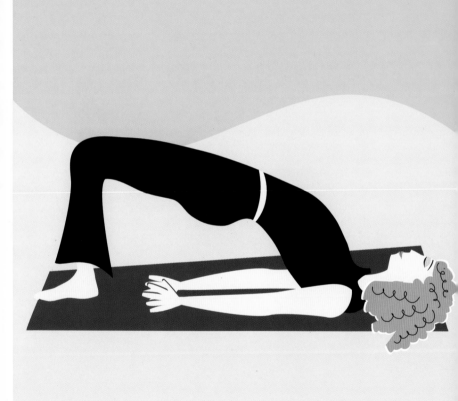

Bridge Pose is a strong and solid posture that strengthens the chest, spine, and neck; revitalizes the legs; calms the mind; reduces stress and fatigue; and expands the chest. Do it as an isolated exercise or as a precursor to Shoulder Stand.

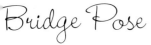

Bridge Pose

* Lie on your back with your knees bent, ankles directly under your knees, feet parallel and hip distance apart.

* Lift your tailbone toward the ceiling, arching your back upward. Your buttocks should be firm but not hard. Your head, neck, and shoulders should remain on the floor.

* Clasp your hands beneath you and stretch your arms toward your feet.

* Lift your buttocks until your thighs are parallel to the floor and then push your tailbone toward your knees. Make sure your knees remain directly over your heels.

* Hold for three breaths and release.

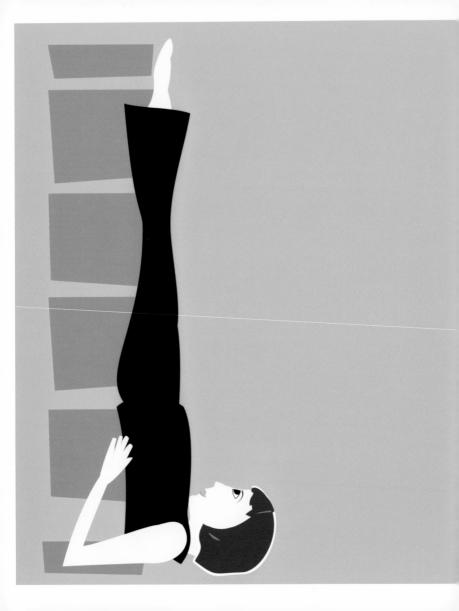

This inversion posture invigorates the entire body. Keep in mind, however, that it is one of the more difficult poses, so take it easy. You may want to start with the Half Shoulder Stand (see the Glow-How below) and work your way up to the full Shoulder Stand. Both postures calm the nervous system, stretch the shoulders and neck, tone the legs and buttocks, strengthen the spine, improve the circulation, and renew energy.

Shoulder Stand

* Lie on your back and bring your knees to your chest. Using your stomach and buttock muscles, curl your hips and legs up in the air.

* Bring your hands to the small of your back for support, fingers facing up, elbows no wider than shoulder width.

* Slowly straighten your legs, pushing your feet up toward the ceiling. Eventually your torso and legs should be in a straight line, perpendicular to the floor.

* Press your shoulders and the backs of your upper arms into the floor for support. Your body weight should be evenly balanced on your shoulders and upper arms.

* Hold for three to five breaths, slowly roll down, and release.

Glow-How

If this posture is too difficult at this point in your practice, try the Half Shoulder Stand. You'll get similar benefits from this pose, but it's a little easier to handle. Begin as you did in full Shoulder Stand, but instead of lifting your legs and torso straight up, lower your hips, moving your hands to your hips for support, and bring your legs back toward your face, holding them about forty-five degrees from the floor.

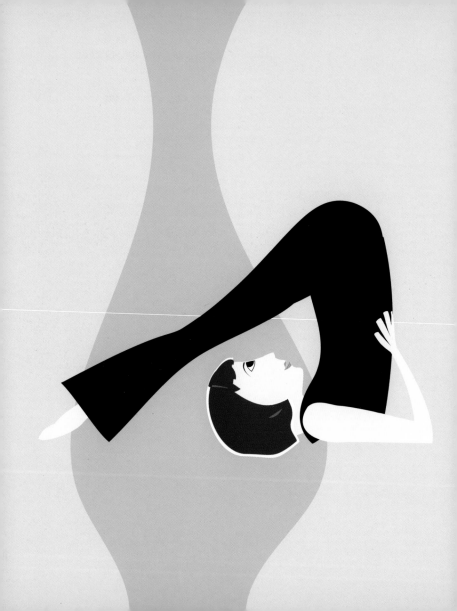

*You can move into this posture directly from Shoulder Stand
or do it independently. Either way, it calms the mind; stimulates
the abdominal organs and thyroid; stretches the shoulders
and spine; tones the abdomen, hips, and legs; strengthens
the nervous system; and improves the circulation.*

Plow

* Lie on your back and bring your knees to
  your chest. Using your stomach and buttocks
  muscles, roll your hips and legs up in the air.

* Bring your hands to the small of your back for
  support, fingers facing up, the back of your
  arms flat on the floor and your elbows close to
  your body.

* Slowly straighten your legs, pushing your feet
  up toward the ceiling.

* Keeping your legs straight, slowly bend from
  the hips, lowering your legs to the floor just
  beyond your head.

* Push your tailbone toward the ceiling, lifting
  your torso. Be sure not to twist your head or neck.

* Hold for three breaths and slowly, in a controlled
  fashion, lift your legs up and roll back down.

Glow-How

This posture
should be done
gracefully. Make
sure your move-
ments flow gently
as you enter and
exit the posture.

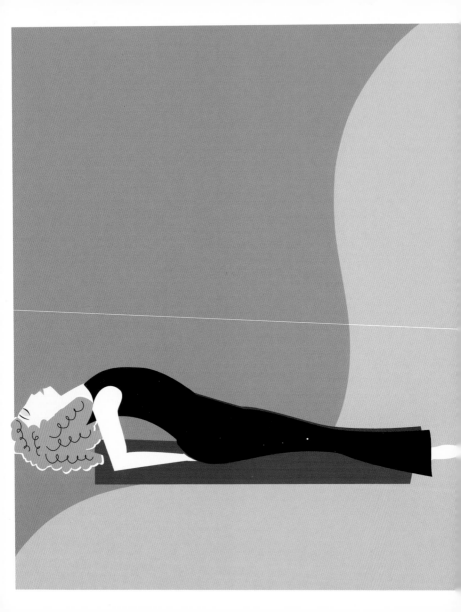

This gentle backward bend is a great counterpose to Plow. It relieves stress and tension, strengthens the neck and spine, and expands the chest.

Fish Pose

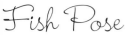

* Lie down on your back with your legs extended straight out in front of you, feet together.

* Bring your arms underneath your body, elbows straight, palms facedown and together, your thumbs touching.

* Lift your chest, arch your back, bring your shoulders together and down, and tilt your head back.

* Support your weight with your arms and elbows as you stretch your legs and slowly lower the top of your head to the floor. There should be very little weight on your head.

* Keep your chest lifted and your legs strong. Hold for three breaths and release.

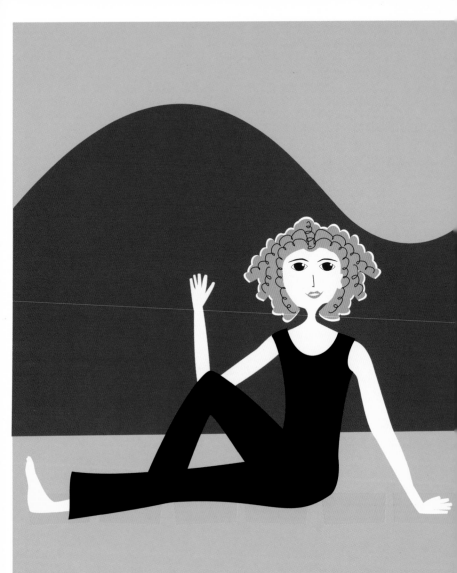

A spinal twist is a great way to wring out toxins from your system, increase the flexibility of your spine, stimulate your internal organs, strengthen your nervous system, and boost your energy. Give it a try when you're feeling a little soggy.

Seated Spinal Twist

* Sit on the floor with your legs extended straight out in front of you.

* Bend your left knee, bringing your left foot over your right leg so that it rests on the outside of your right knee.

* Turn your torso to the left. Place your left hand on the ground next to you, arm straight. Bend your right arm at the elbow, bringing the elbow to the outside of your left knee.

* Keeping your back straight and your shoulders down, lift your chest, stretch your spine, and slowly, gently twist to the left. Use your right elbow as a leverage point, pushing it against your left knee. Turn your head to the left.

* Hold for three to five breaths, release, and switch sides.

Kapalabhati breathing is a powerful respiratory cleansing exercise that also restores energy, strengthens the abdominal muscles and the diaphragm, and improves the circulation. Try it whenever you feel the need to purge yourself of toxic thoughts or emotions. It will help clean out your mind and body with a few quick blasts.

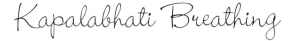

Kapalabhati Breathing

* Take a few normal breaths through your nose.

* After you've taken a moment to get comfortable, inhale as you normally would but, this time, exhale strongly and forcefully. Your nose should make noise as you push out the air and your stomach muscles should contract. Pause for a second.

* Slowly and deeply inhale and, again, exhale sharply, quickly emptying your lungs with a burst of air. Pause for a moment.

* Repeat cycle five times.

Mixing It Up

The purpose of stringing a bunch of postures together—creating a sequence—is to stretch and strengthen the entire body, from head to toe, inside and out. Creating a sequence is actually pretty simple. There's really only one steadfast criterion: Make sure the postures are balanced—follow a backward bend with a forward bend, a deep inhalation with a deep exhalation, the left side with the right side, stretching with contracting, inverted with upright. Get the idea? You're working toward a more balanced body, and a more balanced you.

Each chapter of this book is designed as a mini-sequence, so if you've got an hour, string two or three chapters together, or if you're pressed for time, simply pull a few postures from one chapter and a few more from another, whatever your schedule will allow.

Make sure your sequence jives with how you're feeling on that particular day. If you're tired, do an energizing sequence. Tense? Go with a more gentle series. The point is, you don't have to stick with the same series of poses; arrange the postures in an order that coincides with your mood and energy level from day to day. And once you're more familiar with the postures, it will be easy to come up with a sequence off the top of your head. Your body will almost naturally gravitate from a backward bend into a forward bend, from the left to the right. You'll see!

Sun Salutation

Glow-How

Practicing a sequence of yoga postures in a fluid, continuous movement can increase your cardiovascular workout. Make sure to repeat the series in a relatively rapid succession if you really want to pick up the beat.

The Sun Salutation is a traditional sequence that has been practiced for centuries. Use it as a guide when creating your own series or adopt it as a warm-up. Notice how well all of the postures are balanced.

This particular sequence is done in a continuous stream of movements called a *vinyasa,* each posture flowing into the next. When crafting your own sequence, you may choose to practice a flow of postures as in the Sun Salutation, or you may elect to isolate each posture; either method is fine.

1. Stand with your feet together and your hands at your chest in prayer position. Make sure you're balanced and centered.

2. Keeping your hands together, raise your arms over your head and arch your body back.

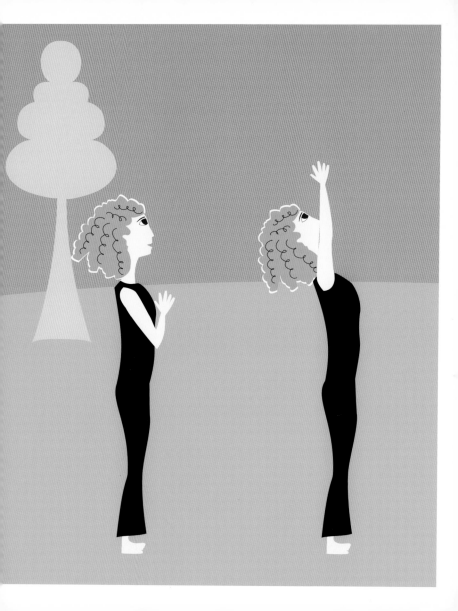

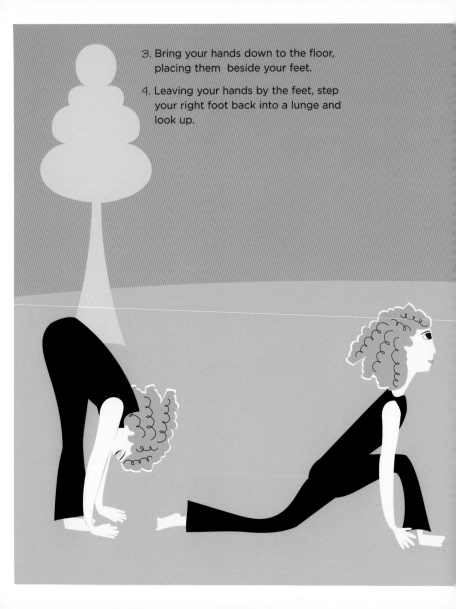

3. Bring your hands down to the floor, placing them beside your feet.

4. Leaving your hands by the feet, step your right foot back into a lunge and look up.

5. Bring your left foot back to meet your right one. Balancing on your toes, keep your arms and legs straight and your back flat.

6. Lift your tailbone slightly as you lower your knees, chest, and chin toward the floor. Push forward and upward as you roll onto the tops of your feet. Lift your chest up, straighten your arms, arch your back, and look up.

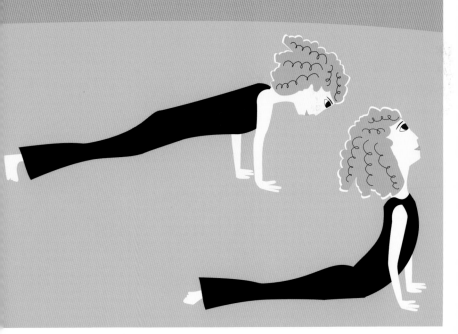

7. Push your hips back and up as you straighten your legs and arms. Press your palms down firmly, engage your thigh muscles, press your heels to the floor, and lengthen your spine.

8. Now step your right foot forward, lunge and look up.

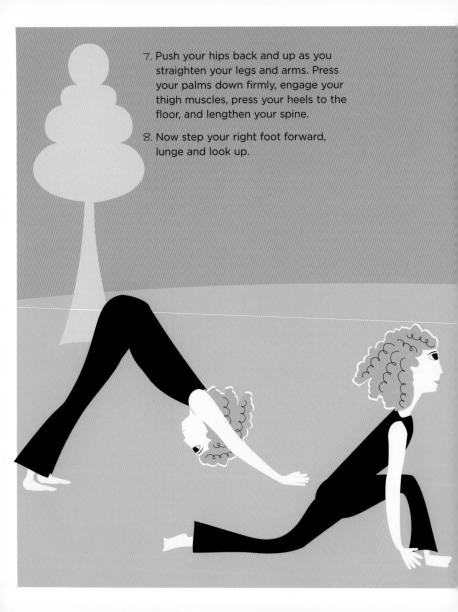

9. Slowly return to the forward bend position and repeat steps 1 and 2.

10. Repeat the series, but this time step back with your left foot.

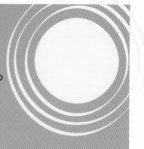

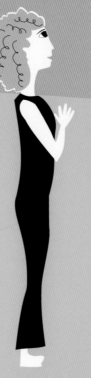

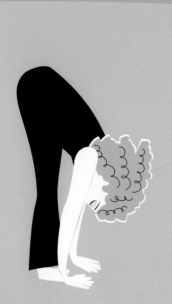

Digging Deeper

Glow Guide: Yoga is designed for beginners and, as such, it really just scratches the surface of the yoga universe. There's a lot more to learn about yoga if you're interested, and the Digging Deeper section was included for that very reason. For those of you who have caught the yoga bug, take a peek at the next few pages. They're full of useful information, including an explanation of various yoga styles, tips on the best way to find a suitable yoga class, suggestions on what you should do (and not do) once you're there, and a list of sources where you can find more information on yoga.

Yoga Styles

Hatha *is the general term used to describe any yoga style in which the primary focus is physical—i.e., the practice of asanas (postures) and pranayama (breath control). This is the type of yoga popular in the West and is what most of us think of when we think: yoga. There are many different approaches to teaching* hatha *yoga out there. Here are the most notable.*

Anusara—Anusara emphasizes the importance of incorporating the spiritual side of yoga into the asana practice. It's more mind-body-spirit oriented than some of the other yoga schools, so if you're not aspiring to achieve supreme consciousness, this one may not be for you.

Ashtanga—One word: hard-core. No yoga flyweights in an ashtanga class. It's a dynamic and vigorous style of yoga and, frankly, the classes (done in a flowing sequence of poses) can be very strenuous, so be prepared to really work.

Bikram—Bikram yoga consists of a series of twenty-six set postures done in a heated room—and the room isn't just warm, it's downright hot. (The temperature of most studios hovers somewhere between 90 and 104 degrees.) This style of yoga is intense, but if you like to sweat—and you *will* sweat—you may want to give it a try.

Intregral—The goal of this yoga is the development of the "complete" individual. This is done through a more slow moving, meditative approach to the practice.

Iyengar—Based on the teachings of the esteemed yoga guru B. K. S. Iyengar, this school is a stickler for alignment and technique. If you want to learn the precise physical alignment of the postures, this may be your class.

Kripalu—Kripalu is a much milder form of yoga geared toward self-discovery. It encourages students to use their practice as a vehicle for self-expression and self-awareness.

Svaroopa—This restorative form of yoga gently works the body to release stress and tension, while also encouraging students to use the time to identify the bad habits or stubborn emotions that may be causing that tension.

Yoga Prescriptions

Aching back? Throbbing head? Yoga to the rescue! Check the listing below for common ailments, and find the yoga poses that can help you overcome them.

Anxiety

Breathing Exercises	33, 50, 68
	86, 104
Bridge Pose	95
Cobbler Pose	80
Sitting Forward Bend	57
Sitting Head-to-Knee Pose	85
Standing Forward Bend	79
Triangle Pose	27

Constipation

Fish Pose	101
Knees-to-Chest Pose	63
Plow	99
Shoulder Stand	97
Sitting Forward Bend	57
Sitting Head-to-Knee Pose	85
Spinal Twists	58, 103
Standing Forward Bend	79

Backache

Half Boat Pose	37
Bow Pose	55
Bridge Pose	95
Cat Pose	92
Cobra Pose	53
Downward-Facing Dog	65
Fish Pose	101
Leg Lifts	21, 83
Lightning Bolt Pose	23
Plow	99
Shoulder Stand	97
Spinal Twists	58, 103
Triangle Pose	27
Wheel Pose	61

Fatigue

Breathing Exercises	33, 50, 68
	86, 104
Bridge Pose	95
Child Pose	75
Cobbler Pose	80
Cobra Pose	53
Downward-Facing Dog	65
Plow	99
Shoulder Stand	97
Sitting Head-to-Knee Pose	85
Standing Forward Bend	79
Upward-Facing Dog	91

Finding the Right Yoga School

First off, it helps to decide what kind of yoga you'd like to do. Are you looking for something mild and more meditative, or perhaps something more aggressive? Once you've narrowed it down, it will be easier to pinpoint the right school for you. If you're not sure, that's okay; you'll just have to do a little studio hopping until you settle on a style that suits your needs.

When it's time to start the actual search, ask your friends, classmates, and coworkers about their yoga schools. Yogis are usually pretty eager to chat with possible recruits. You can also consult your local Yellow Pages; it will list many of the studios in your area. Or check out the three Web sites listed in the Yoga Resource Guide. Each one hosts a national directory of schools. Pick out a few and give them each a call.

Here are a few questions to ask:

- * What type of yoga do you teach?
- * How long are the classes?
- * What class should I take if I'm a beginner?
- * What should I wear?
- * How much does it cost?
- * Do I need to bring my own mat and towel or do you provide them?
- * Do you have a changing room?
- * Can you send me a class schedule?

Now narrow down your list to a few choice studios. Give each class a try and see what suits you the best. Once you've settled on a school, it's usually a good idea to continue going to that school. This gives the teachers a chance to become familiar with your needs and limitations, so they can help you get the most out of the classes.

Classroom Etiquette and Other Important Stuff

Don't eat for at least two hours before class. A full stomach will disrupt your yoga flow and may make you feel sick.

Drink lots of water the day of your class. Sure, you can bring water into class (though at some studios it's frowned upon), but it is better to be hydrated before you show up.

If possible, bike or walk to the studio. This will increase your circulation and help get your body warmed up for class.

Don't wear perfume or any scented lotions to class. It can distract or offend the other students.

Arrive early. This will give you some extra time to sign in, pay, change, and get familiar with the place.

Apprise your teacher of any old injuries or particular conditions that may affect your practice. This way the teacher can help you modify certain postures if necessary.

During class, don't talk. This is distracting to others and to the teacher.

Shed any worries about looking funny. For the most part, people are so focused on their postures, they won't even notice you.

Don't compare yourself to other students. Everyone's practice is different—focus on your own.

Take it easy the first few classes. Let your body get used to the yoga before you start to really push it. You don't want to strain or injure yourself right out of the gates.

It's best not to enter the classroom late, leave early, or walk in and out during class. This can be highly distracting to the other students.

When class is over, give yourself a few moments of still-ness before leaping up and running off to your next engagement. Allow your body the opportunity to soak in the effects of the yoga.

Thank yourself for showing up and sticking it out!

Yoga Resource Guide

Popular yoga magazines:
Yoga Journal
Yoga International

On-line resources teeming with yoga info:
www.yogadirectory.com
www.yogasite.com
www.yogajournal.com

Sites devoted to specific styles of yoga:
www.anusara.com
www.ashtanga.com
www.bikramyoga.com
www.bksiyengar.com
www.kripalu.org
www.masteryoga.org (Svaroopa)
www.yogaville.org (Intregral)

**Other illustrated yoga guides
from Chronicle Books:**
Om Yoga: A Guide to Daily Practice by Cyndi Lee, 2002
Office Yoga: Simple Stretches for Busy People
   by Darrin Zeer, 2000
*The Yoga Deck: 50 Poses & Meditations for Body,
   Mind & Spirit* by Olivia H. Miller, 2002